MW01257310

7 Stages of Teeth presents

Denture Adventure

The year I got teeth
for my birthday

Table of Contents

To Rick, my amazing husband and faithful denture adventure co-pilot. I couldn't have done it without you. And to Dick, and Deb, for all their long-distance support. You gave me strength.

About This Book

This book was born from my frustration. When I was considering dentures, I wanted to know everything I could about the process. I hate feeling out of control. Knowledge is power, as they say, and I wanted to know it all. What I found online didn't answer all my questions. I wanted to know what to expect – everything, from the procedure itself to how to put the teeth in and how it worked to eat with them.

Most of the information I found online was general instructions on how to eat – chew on both sides, take small bites. There were also general instructions on keeping the dentures secure, and cleaning the dentures – brought to you from the manufacturers of each particular product. I wanted something more personal. I definitely wanted something more than a commercial for a particular dentist or manufacturer.

I found some YouTube videos that were helpful. One brave young man actually showed how he put his teeth in every morning. The normalcy of it all was tremendously reassuring. Another video was a woman who recorded herself after a procedure. She spoke about the procedure and how easily it went. Her mouth was bleeding a bit; she paused at regular intervals to sip water, then went on speaking about how she was feeling. I watched, fascinated. Here was an "ordinary" person, someone who had actually been through the process.

She helped me feel calmer. I wish I could remember her name, or the name of the young man who showed how to insert dentures. If I could, I would thank them.

I have never been one to record my thoughts on video. As a writer, words have always been my outlet. So here are my thoughts, in diary form, of my "denture adventure". I hope you find them useful.

"What are the 7 Stages of Teeth?"

Getting dentures was an experience, to say the least! As I went through the process, I discovered that there were 7 distinct stages. These are not neat, in-numerical-orderly stages. In the first four or five weeks, I experienced some of them multiple times.

Here is a brief summary of each stage:

STAGE 1 - "Chew on This" – Decisions, decisions - Research comforts me, allowing me to apply reason and logic to an emotional time. So many questions: Who should I go to? What will it be like? How do you put dentures in? The anxiety of realizing I can't put this off any longer. Then - feeling pressured, the decision to get a second opinion. The research stage gets repeated each time I have a new question or concern.

STAGE 2 - "Numb-founded" - Relief – it's over, I made it. Twenty (20) extractions and the placement of immediate dentures in one visit; bloodied and battle-scarred, still numb from the drugs. Can't feel my face or lips or nose. It might hurt. I think it Does hurt, in fact. But the magic pain pills make me numb to it all. Can't feel anything but relief right now. I drift. And sleep a lot.

STAGE 3 - "Smiley face"- Filled with wonder and awe - Hey look! I have teeth! Cool! Selfie time! I have to learn how to smile all over again. For years I have been avoiding a full smile, trying to keep my lips together. It feels odd to include my teeth. I look in the mirror and say "cheese".

STAGE 4 - "Bite Me!" - Anger/Frustration - Why is this taking so long? Why does it still hurt? And why on earth do I need more goop in my mouth? I hate dentures! I feel like a freak! Angry at everyone. Potato chips defeat me.

STAGE 5 - "Eating is a Bother"- Depression - No end in sight. Feels like this frustration will never end. I lose interest in food. Not worth the effort. "I'm not hungry," I tell my husband. "Eating is a bother."

STAGE 6 - "Fear me Food!" Determination - I Will conquer and rise above this challenge. My rebellious streak is coming out. Nobody is going to tell me I can't eat that! I attack a pancake and win! Taste doesn't enter in to the equation. It's all about crushing the enemy - food!

STAGE 7 - "Teeth Truce" Acceptance - I am becoming accustomed to dentures. There are whole minutes when I forget I have them. To quote Eeyore the Donkey, "it ain't much of a tail but I'm kind of attached to it. Store bought is better than nothing.

Week 1 - And then there were none

(**FEB 5TH, 2015**; "D-Day" and B-Day – My 61st Birthday) Stage 2 – "Relief". "TGIO! - "Thank God It's Over"! Relief is definitely the first stage after the event. I had been given Valium to take prior to the procedure - 1 tablet the night before, then 2 tablets an hour before the appointment. They called this "conscious sedation".

Supposedly I would be so relaxed that I might not even remember all of the procedure and it would seem like it went faster. Wrong! I was quite alert, and way too conscious. The Valium just seemed to make me a bit woozy and unable to resist. I would definitely ask for something stronger if I had it to do all over again. I chose the pills over gas because I had read that nitrous oxide (commonly known as "laughing gas") could cause nausea, and I hate throwing up.

They also advised me to bring music so I had my iPod with me. But the music wasn't loud enough. I could hear crunching sounds as the dentist pulled my teeth. The noise was so loud that it all but drowned out my favorite Jimmy Buffett song, "Breathe In, Breathe Out Move On". I tried to turn the music up but it was hard to reach my iPod, and impossible to see the controls from my prone position. So I just tried to listen harder. There were also some teeth that seemed to resist being pulled. I could feel the dull tugging sensation. One tooth was infected, a fact that became clear when they tried to extract it.

The unexpected pain caused me to raise my hand - the signal the dentist had arranged if I needed him to stop. He apologized for hurting me and explained that they couldn't know the tooth was infected till they 'got in there'. They gave me more injections of Novocain, and left me for a few minutes while it took effect. My face already felt like a bloated, weeks-dead carp washed up on a beach. And It still hurt; infected areas can't be numbed (as I learned later).

By this point, the drugs and my patience were both waning, and I just wanted the nightmare to be over. I used my alone time to turn up the volume on my iPod and do some deep breathing. Then I shut my eyes, opened my mouth and lay back.

The dentist might have known there was an infected tooth had the receptionist not lost my complete x-rays. This also meant I had to get a quick retake before the procedure could begin. Full x-rays had been taken by the previous dentist I went to just two weeks prior.

That office had emailed them to my new dentist and apparently they were lost during some computer upgrade. I try not to judge but - really guys? This wasn't helping my stress level. I have an extreme dental phobia. For years, my mouth would automatically clamp shut at the mere mention of a dentist. I staunchly refused to go see anyone, preferring to just ignore the problem as long as possible. When at last I accepted that something had to be done, I wanted it done quickly, before I could come up with any more excuses. This was my biggest fear – and I had faced it! I felt an overwhelming feeling of relief mixed with wonder. I did it! Yay, me.

One note in hindsight - choosing to do this on my birthday was probably Not the smartest thing. When I set up the appointment, I told the receptionist it was my birthday. She joked about how, afterward, I'd be able to eat steak and pizza. I probably should have clarified how long "after" - because it sure sounded pretty immediate! Then there was that term - "immediate dentures". It all sounded so fast and easy. I don't think dentists realize, how uninformed we are when we go there. "Ask questions", they tell us. And I want to say "what questions do I have?"

There are things I know now, that I should have asked. But that is now. So the one piece of advice I would offer dentists is - tell us. Everything. What you are going to do, what it will feel or taste like, and please, please - maybe some suggestions for coping! My advice to patients is similar. Ask the dentist to explain everything. Let them know if you are scared to the point of paralysis. You aren't the first to feel that way.

Donna Wylie

(FEB 6TH, 2015; 1 day after the procedure) Stage 3 - "Smiley face"- Still drugged but awake enough to post to Facebook. Picture of my new look:

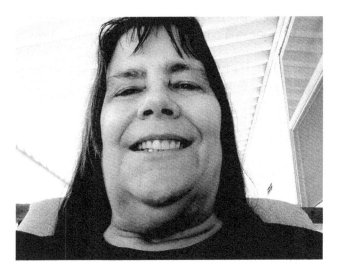

I don't post the "before" look. Too embarrassed. Haven't smiled in pictures in years.

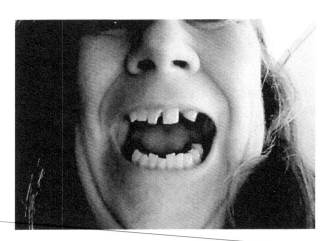

Denture Adventure

(FEB 7TH, 2015) 2 days after the procedure, still on pain meds. I am now supposed to take the teeth out 3 - 4 times a day to clean them. Of course I was not given any instructions on how to do this. When I called the dentist the (new) receptionist told me to refer to the sheet they had given me after the procedure. The sheet was about tooth extractions. Single. Not multiple teeth and dentures. I tried to tell the girl that I didn't see any instructions for my situation. She condescendingly suggested I have my husband look at the sheet. I presume this was because he had accompanied me to the appointment and she assumed I was so drugged up on Vicodin that what? I couldn't read?

I finally gave up and googled what to do. They also hadn't given me a case for the dentures. Thank god for plastic containers. I rinsed the dentures in plain water and rinsed my mouth with warm salt water. This was something else I didn't learn from the dentist. My father-in-law (who also has dentures) had been following my progress closely, and he suggested the rinse. Google agreed – salt is a natural disinfectant and helps reduce swelling. Kind of taking the whole "DIY" thing to the extreme. But one thing I won't do is piss off someone who is still in charge of my mouth! So I don't complain.

I decide I am coherent enough (I think) to take a shower. My first since the procedure. Getting out of the tub, I feel a wave a dizziness and nausea. No wonder, Rick says, when I tell him about it later. All I have eaten for two days is soup, yogurt, gelatin and pudding. Ah yes, the denture diet! I do Not recommend it!

Rick spends a lot of time and effort finding me food I can eat that is more nutritious. He makes packaged mashed potatoes and puts gravy over top. Tastes like heaven!

Amazing how good food is when you haven't been able to eat it.

(FEB. 8, 2015) Stage 4 - And then there was pain.... The day started well. I woke feeling good and Rick said my face was less swollen. Yay, I thought. The worst is over. Wrong. The afternoon brought an attack of pain in my sinuses. My whole face hurt. Vicodin didn't help. Cold cloth, a dark room and a warm Chihuahua help dull the pain somewhat.

(FEB 9, 2015) My face feels swollen. Rick says it looks puffy. Still a lot of sinus pain. A Facebook friend tells me it must be an infection. She says I should be on antibiotics and that the dentist should be able to prescribe them over the phone. It sounds logical. I had asked about pre-procedure antibiotics since I have a prolapsed mitral valve in my heart and they used to advise antibiotics before any medical procedure. Of course that was decades ago. And the receptionist (an experienced one - I think) had told me they no longer do that. Still, after everything they had messed up I was feeling less than confident so

Denture Adventure

I emailed the dentist office, explained about my sinus pain and asked about antibiotics.

The woman responds an infection is "unlikely." I feel as though I have insulted them somehow. She says the dentist will need to see me before he prescribes anything and sets me up with an appointment for the following day. We do accomplish one thing - we finally get the message across that I have no information on what to do with my dentures as far as cleaning, storage etc.

I again explain that the instruction sheet I was given was for a single tooth extraction, with no mention of dentures. I say I think they forgot to give me the denture information. She replies that they didn't forget, she just wrote up the instructions and will email them to me. Rick and I are dumb-founded. At this point we are both wondering if these people have ever done dentures before! My father-in-law goes to this dentist for his dentures. Plus, the dentist has his own lab where he makes the dentures. And I love the dentist. He is kind and caring and reassuring. But the staff gets a "F" for communication.
The instruction sheet we finally receive confirms what I have already discovered online as far as care.

(FEB 10, 2015) Back at the dentist, two days early for my follow-up appointment. The doctor says everything looks good, I just have some pressure sores in my mouth. He is going to adjust the dentures he says and they should feel

Donna Wylie

a lot better afterward. He tells me to keep the
dentures out for the next three days to allow
my gums to heal. After that, I should remove the
dentures at night. He makes an appointment for
a week later, says he will do the soft reline at that
time and how 'that should really make a difference.' Again, the fault is mine, possibly, for not
clarifying if it would be pleasant. Also, as it turns
out, we have two diverse concepts of what "soft"
means. I go home happy to have an end (I think)
in sight, happily anticipating some sort of
malleable material for the new reline.

Rick makes me boxed macaroni & cheese, using a
potato masher to make the pieces smaller. I
nearly wept with joy when I tasted it! "Real
food!", I exclaimed.

It may sound absurd but when all you have
been eating is soup, gelatin, pudding and yogurt,
anything with texture is pure wonderment.
Rick adds in more foods - tuna fish with plenty
of mayo; steamed cauliflower that I mash with
butter and salt and pepper; fish that can be flaked
and mashed; canned green beans; meat-loaf.

Anything that can be mashed or broken into
small enough pieces to swallow. As Rick points
out, "most people don't chew their food anyway."
He's given this a lot of thought.

Week 2 - 2 bites forward, 1 step back

(**FEB 13, 2015**) Pain. Still on Vicodin, still experiencing mouth sores, still feeling angry.

(**FEB 15, 2015**) My father-in-law has been more help than the staff at the dentist's office. He has kept in touch with Rick, checking on my progress, both before and after the procedure. It helped me tremendously, to know how much he cared. His suggestions, like rinsing with salt water, and his stories about his own experiences with dentures, really helped me feel less alone.

My husband has been nothing short of amazing! Last night he told me something I hadn't known. He said that first night, after the procedure, he stayed awake the whole night, watching over me. He was worried about how much I was bleeding, and said he wanted to make sure I wasn't going to hemorrhage or anything.

The dentist had told us to expect a "little oozing" after the procedure; this seemed more like a flood! It took several hours and a roll of gauze, for the blood to slow to the point where it could be considered a minor "ooze".

Rick has also been doing all the cooking, working to find foods I could eat and enjoy. He spent multiple hours wandering the grocery store, searching every aisle for food that would be easy to eat.

Donna Wylie

Today my mouth hurts a little less and I was off the Vicodin while my teeth were out. I had been instructed by the dentist, to take the teeth out at night, to give my mouth time to heal. But when I put the teeth back in Thursday morning, it felt like the uppers were going to fall out. They were so loose! It took three tries to get them in and settled!

I still struggle with depression. This has been such a major adjustment. I am back on Vicodin, but at a reduced amount, just one or two times a day.

I do take the teeth out to eat, but I am trying to adjust to eating with them in. I ate my breakfast with them in – scrambled eggs with ham bits. Still can't chew. The bottom teeth are too loose and hurt if I press on them. Plus, it feels like I am trying to swallow around a mouthful of – well – teeth!

As Rick and I discussed last night, this could have gone a lot worse. I haven't had any dry sockets, the pain has been tolerable, and I have had lots of support. My younger sister, Deb, has also been great about keeping in touch by text, checking to see how I am feeling.

Deb also shared her experience with a single-tooth implant. It was reassuring to hear how long she took to heal. Like my father-in-law, my sister's stories helped me feel more "normal" and less alone.Since I had never been through this process before, I had no idea what was normal or expected. Dentists do this stuff so often that they forget how terrifyingly unfamiliar all this can be to their patients. My sister observed that dentists don't understand how their patients feel, because they haven't had oral surgery. I replied maybe that should be a requirement, to get their license! If only!

(FEB 17, 2015) Yuck! Not a good dental visit! The soft reline material smelled and tasted like shellac! I tried to use techniques from when I had the impressions made. That experience was awful but endurable. The woman who did it warned me it would be unpleasant. And she gave me coping techniques - sit forward if it makes you gag. Count. March in place, moving your feet as you march and counting so you can focus on something other than that tray of goop in your mouth! She also gave me power to choose. Did I want the most difficult one (uppers) first? Or last?

Such choices helped me feel more in control. The reline material is more challenging for me. Unlike the impression material, it seemed to take forever to set. When the dentist first put the dentures in my mouth and I tasted the awful taste, I started shaking. A panic attack, perhaps. The doctor told me to clench my teeth together and hold it for 'a few minutes'. I was shaking so hard my teeth were chattering, and the dentist said "No. You need to keep your jaws together."

Donna Wylie

Matter of fact. Like it was that easy. Easier said than done, I want to reply, but I'm not allowed to open my mouth. I finally manage to keep my teeth together but it took all my strength and willpower to get through those few minutes.

The dentist had warned me that the reline material "didn't taste very good" – a definite understatement! I should have known. After all, this was the same man who told me to expect a "little oozing" after my teeth were pulled. I held on by focusing on the fact that this was all temporary. Just have to get through the next few minutes; one more song on my iPod; count to 60 five times. Having my husband there with me was my saving grace. Rick kept up a steady stream of reassurances, telling me how good I was doing, how it was almost over. True or not, his voice was the calming anchor I clung to, like a rock in a stormy sea.

The dentist came back in to check on me once or twice. One time he asked if I was okay and I shook my head emphatically. No! He patted my shoulder and told me to hang in there. My husband told him I looked like I was going to be sick. My face was a ghostly white, Rick told me afterward. He had already checked for where the wastebasket was in case I needed to throw up.

The dentist came and took the teeth to trim the lining. I rinsed my mouth repeatedly but couldn't seem to get the taste to go away. At least the

Denture Adventure

worst was over, I thought. I was wrong! I had assumed the awful tasting glop was temporary, like the impressions material. Wrong again! The awful tasting glop was the reline material!

The dentist came back and put the teeth in my mouth, telling me to push them in further. They now fit more securely in my mouth. I was told to come back in 10 – 14 days. Meanwhile I should try to keep the teeth in, and eat with them. I asked if I should still remove the teeth at night, and the dentist said yes. He added that I could remove them whenever I needed to. I thought that was a bit odd...until we left the office.

 As we walked to the car, I started to gag and retch. The dentist had asked if I had a water bottle in the car. He had told me the taste of the reline would go away and advised me to rinse. I composed myself and we continued to the parking lot. When we got to the car, I sat a few minutes. I rinsed my mouth a several times, spitting the water into the parking lot. Finally, I took the teeth out, and wrapped them in napkins I dampened with water. Then we drove home.

I kept the teeth out the rest of the day, soaking them in a bath of baking soda and water. I had found that suggestion online. There had been no instructions from the dentist. It's easy to look back and say, I could have just asked. But at the time, when I was feeling gaggy and stressed, I wasn't thinking clearly. The taste had been a shock, along the knowledge that it was now part

of my permanent teeth. This morning, I
brushed my mouth with toothpaste and rinsed
with mouthwash. Feeling at least partly prepared, I inserted the top teeth. I immediately
began gagging. I pulled the plate back out,
feeling frustrated.

Stubbornly, I tried again, this time starting with
the lowers. I had a slight gag response, but
focused on breathing through my nose slowly, to
calm myself. Gingerly, I tried inserting the upper
plate again. This time the gag reflex wasn't as bad
and I managed to keep the teeth in my mouth.
I had my usual cup of coffee. Swallowing is hard.
The back edge of my upper plate scrapes against
my tongue. I find I can control that somewhat by
putting my tongue forward and pressing firmly
against the upper plate. Gonna try pancaked for
breakfast. Wish me luck!

A word about my faithful "denture co-pilot",
my husband, Rick. He was there by my side for
every appointment, reading to me, rubbing my
back, calming me with his presence. I don't know
how I would have made it through without him.
If you have such a person in your life, don't be
afraid to ask them for help.

The potent taste and smell of the reline material
is supposed to fade "after a few days," according
to what I read online. Those few days seemed
to last for weeks! The dentist told me the reline
would make the dentures fit better so I could
start eating more solid food. Almost two weeks

after the procedure. It seems a lifetime has passed. Why is it taking so long? IS this long? The doctor also said something about six months until my gums are 'settled'. Or something. Do I have to wait that long to eat regular food? I feel angry, frustrated, depressed.

(FEB 18, 2015) My sister Deb suggests adding a pinch of ground cloves to the baking soda and water soak. The spice is a natural pain reliever; plus, the smell and taste might overpower the reline odor. I try that the next night, with some success. Now the reline tastes like spicy shellac! Hindsight tip—if you try this you should probably use clove oil instead of ground cloves. The ground cloves powder dissolved and turned the soak water brown. It Could have stained the teeth. Fortunately, I woke early, thinking of that very likelihood, and 'rescued' the teeth.

Rick makes pancakes for breakfast so I can try chewing with my new teeth. Slow going! As my research instructed, I cut everything into small bites and try to chew with the back teeth, on both sides at once. Since I never ate like this to begin with, it seems to take forever. Can't remember if I even tasted anything, I was so busy focusing on chewing. End result? I'm thinking maybe soft food isn't so bad.

(FEB 19, 2015) Feeling depressed. "Eating is such a bother", I tell Rick. I have my morning coffee but nothing else, even though Rick offers to make me scrambled eggs. I just don't feel breakfast-y", I tell Rick. My terminology makes him laugh. We go to the town library. This is our first visit since moving to Mesa in December 2014. We spend time browsing a book sale, checking out books, and getting library cards. The familiar routine of getting settled in a new city is comforting. I'm beginning to feel like we belong here. Driving home, I realize I am feeling woozy and sick to my stomach, the result of not eating breakfast.

(FEB 20, 2015) I test out actually biting food. My first experiment - pancake with jelly. Yes, just one. Eating is a long process; so I take it in (literally!) baby steps. A friend had warned me "you have to learn to eat all over again." At the time, I had no idea what that really meant or what would be involved!

Learning to eat evokes a myriad of feelings - frustration, anger, determination and depression. Depression was the most pervasive feeling. But there was also loneliness. Or more appropriately, a feeling of aloneness.

Conversely, there is also joy and triumph. A sense of accomplishment over the simple act of biting and chewing. I feel a silly smugness - Ha! Stupid teeth! Take that, evil pancake! Then just as quickly, I am back to anger and resentment. The feelings shifted so quickly that I was left feeling exhausted, like I had been through Tropical Storm "Manic-Depressive"!But, hey - I did it! I'm proud of myself. I have conquered the scary

Denture Adventure

pancake! I am a food warrior! Fear me, pancake!
Then, boom I am back to doubt and frustration. I
think of eating pizza and it overwhelms me. How
many bite-steps down the road is that prize? Food
Warrior rises up. No! I won't think of the future!
Like a 12-stepper, I will focus on just this bite.
And celebrate each small step.

Another step. Sideways I think. Inspired by my
pancake feat, I try a tuna "sandwich" for lunch.
Rick makes a bowl of well - mayonnaised tuna,
and gives me a slice of white bread. I tear off the
crusts, put a small forkful of tuna on one corner
and bite. No go. I am afraid to bite with the front
teeth. Thought I read somewhere that I should
use the back ones. Can that be right? The back
ones are more for chewing, not biting. I try again.
Clamp down on the bread and tear off the small
piece. Once in my mouth the tuna and bread
feels huge! Unwieldy. It slides on the slick surface
of my upper plate, heading for my throat like a
runaway roller coaster. I manage to stop it by
gagging it forward. Not sure that was intentional
but it works. I roll the bite around until I can get it
to the back teeth to 'chew'. Although at this point
that is hardly necessary, I feel a stubborn need to
dominate the squishy bundle. I swallow. One bite
down. Ye gods, I think. At this rate lunch could
take me until supper-time to consume. I switch
to a more practical approach, tearing bits of bread
into my bowl, I spear them along with some tuna
and place the forkful into the back my mouth.
It still feels as if I am just 'going through the
motions' of eating. Literally! I am relieved when I

Donna Wylie

manage to finish the task.

Week 3 - Are we there yet?

(FEB 21, 2015) Today I try a turkey burger and tater tots for lunch. Hamburger would have been a better choice as far as texture. Or a hand-made turkey burger. Something less resistant to my need to pre-mash everything. I will keep that in mind for next time.

Rick cooks the patty to the recommended internal temp, always looking out for my safety. Had I cooked it myself, I would have under-done it. That has always been my preference, even 'Pre-D'. I liked the softer texture. But no matter. I resolve to conquer this new challenge.
I cut the patty into small bites, no larger than maybe ½ inch square. I also dice up the tater tots and add enough ketchup to make them moist. I use my fork to place tiny bites in the back of my mouth. I can't feel the food and so I chew a bit then swallow. It's a frustratingly slow process.

Eating has become a chore that I dread. Like practicing scales on a piano, or reciting times tables, it is the tedium I must endure to get where I want to be--a concert chew-ist! I fear I will never succeed. But I persevere, telling myself that this too shall pass. Please, God, let this pass! We take a drive to a park where we walk a bit and take pictures. A nice break. On the way home, we stop for ice cream at my request. A cone sounds good. Soft serve from Dairy Queen. I manage it quite nicely. I can't take bites of the pointed top of the ice cream--it feels strange when I open my mouth too wide. So I just lick. It tastes good and I am feeling content until....I come to the cone. Damn! There is still ice cream. Quite a bit of it in fact. My life-long habit has always been to push the ice cream into the cone as I ate. Avoids drips that way. And I love the taste of an ice-cream moistened cone. There is only one problem. I can't figure out how to bite the cone.

Fortunately, we are close to home, where I finish getting the ice cream out with a spoon. It isn't ideal but it works. I could break up the cone to 'chew' it that way. But it just isn't the same as how I Used to be able to eat. I can't take dainty bites, making the cone last, savoring it all the way to the last bite. Depressed, I discard the empty cone. For supper, I choose easy - fish fillet and boxed mac and cheese. Both chopped up into easily-swallowed bits. I am tired of trying to learn to eat and don't want to try any more today.

(**FEB 22, 2015**) I go with 'easy' for breakfast. Graham crackers in milk. Childhood comfort food. I'm not ready to face reality just yet. It feels like I am going backwards.

Suppertime - A momentous occasion, according to Rick. My 1st time eating chicken! We got a whole cooked chicken from the grocery store, and used just the breast meat for supper. Rick diced my portion finely, and I ate it over mashed potatoes with gravy. Pure heaven! The meat was tender enough that it didn't offer any resistance to my novice chewing attempts. I ate two helpings!

(FEB 23, 2015) I come up with a great supper idea, using the leftover meat from last night's chicken. I grind the meat in my food processor - fast and easy. I get about 1 ½ cups ground. Then I mix in a generous amount of shredded Mexican blend sharp cheese (about 1 cup), along with some pizza blend shredded cheese (about ¼ cup). A tablespoon of taco sauce (could probably forgo that next time - it's spicy enough with the enchilada sauce). And a heaping tablespoon of sour cream. I add ¾ cup of enchilada sauce and mix everything together.
I use ¼ cup of enchilada sauce to "grease" the baking dish, and preheat the oven to 350 degrees. I put a heaping tablespoon of chicken mix on a corn tortilla and roll it up, placing seam side down in the prepared pan. Makes about 6 generously filled rolls.

I cover everything with more enchilada sauce and sprinkle another ¼ cup or so of cheese over the top. Cover with foil and bake for 35 - 40 minutes until heated through. Serve with generous dollop of sour cream.
Could add a side of refried beans, and maybe some sliced avocado. Rick says yuck to the avocado, but he raves about the enchiladas! It almost feels like a "normal" meal! The great benefit of using corn tortillas is that they get soft very

easily. So even without teeth, they present no challenge. The variations are endless. Could add well-cooked rice, refried beans, different meat, etc.!

(FEB 24, 2015) Lunch is a bean and cheese enchilada - refried beans and shredded cheese on corn tortillas, rolled up and covered with enchilada sauce. Cover with foil, bake at 350 degrees for about 25 minutes. Serve with sour cream and sliced avocado. Yummy!
For supper, we try out some small pasta that (in theory) should be easier to eat. Ditalini, Italian for "small thimbles", is a type of pasta that is shaped like small tubes. We give it a try. Nothing fancy, just pasta and spaghetti sauce. The sauce is Hunts brand – it comes in cans and is less expensive than the bottled sauces. It also has no 'lumps' - a pleasant surprise! We will definitely use that brand in the future!

This kind of meal is also familiar and comfortingly normal. We love pasta and sauce. We have never liked the lumps of tomatoes in spaghetti sauce or salsa. Rick has gone so far as to puree salsa when he wants a snack of chips and salsa. I know that may sound odd. But we want the flavor blended, not in chunks. Which is why I substitute taco sauce for salsa in my 'toothless' meals. So back to the pasta. I thought the smaller shapes would be easier but instead they seem to get 'lost' in my mouth, slipping down my throat before I can catch them with my inexperienced teeth. In the future, I would either use standard spaghetti that can be cut up, or smaller shapes that can be swallowed - perhaps small rings, similar to those found in canned pasta.

(FEB 25, 2015) Another momentous occasion! I conquered Frosted Flakes! (It's the little things). Too hungry to wait for the milk to make them soggy, I dive right in. Throwing caution to the wind, I chew. Hurrah for me! AND - I did it with dentures that are a bit on the loose side since I am due for another adjustment tomorrow. This is no easy feat, since it requires careful balancing of the food on my teeth so as to not rock the dentures. Keeping them securely in my mouth is vital for preventing food bits from getting stuck under the teeth. I smile. I think I may eventually learn to eat with these things! They still give me a gaggy feeling sometimes. And I am still getting those 'back of the head' sinus headaches. Hopefully this too shall pass as both my mind and mouth get used to these new teeth.

Tomorrow is the 3-week anniversary of my new teeth! (wonder if there will be cake?) NOT looking forward to the dentist. And possibly another reline. Gonna try a Valium before I go, maybe that will help. Last time caught me off-guard and unprepared! I have no idea how many more visits it will take, or what will need to be done before I can do just the normal twice yearly appointments. Going to look for someone closer to home once I am through with the denture stuff. Too many issues with this place. Not the dentist, who is great, but his staff. Their

Donna Wylie

mistakes have been too frequent for my comfort. The latest error? - a bill that is $500 - $600 More than the original quote! Reason? They 'forgot' to list all the teeth that were being removed! The original invoice had 14 teeth listed. The bill says 20! Then there is the matter of 20 not being correct either! The first dentist had planned to leave 4 anchor teeth on the bottom and quoted me for extraction of 17 teeth. This dentist left just 2 anchor teeth. So how does 17 + 2 = 20? Yup, if there was a way to switch now I would!

(FEB 26, 2015) Just back from the dentist. My feelings go back and forth on them. They are all so nice it's hard to be angry at them. We got the bill explained – the additional tooth was just a root tip. Okay - I'll give them that. The original estimate of 14 extractions, though, that had the office manager stumped! And speechless. I think she was afraid I was going to tell her to knock that extra $600 off the bill since it's their error. With the billing questions answered, it was time to get on with the reline.

The dental assistant removed the soft reline from the first time and did a new fitting, just on my top plate. The dentist called it a "gum conditioner" when I said reline. Apparently a reline is different? The taste was just as gag-awful as the first time. But the experience was not as bad as the first time. The assistant is better at applying the paste, I think. She also stayed and talked me through the process, instead of just telling me to "hang in there".

Denture Adventure

Carrie (the assistant) told me to breathe through my nose, and demonstrated what she meant. I followed her lead and immediately felt calmer and more in control. I was already following her advice to lean forward. The dentist stopped by and told me to put my feet on the floor so I could lean forward farther. Those suggestions, combined with Carrie's soothing chairside manner, got me through the process with a minimum of stress.

So a couple tips - lean forward and focus on breathing through your nose slowly. Also, don't forget to charge your iPod! My batteries were dead, which meant my calming music was not available, and that made me panic. So be prepared. Here's where a denture co-pilot comes in handy (watch for this and other tips in our soon-to-be-released booklet – "I'm with Toothless – A Guide for Denture Co-Pilots").

I have a request for all dentists: Don't (please, do Not!) discuss the procedure with your assistant while you are in the same room as a patient who is struggling not to vomit! Phrases like how "goopy" the mixture should be, and how it should "ooze out the sides" and not be "runny"? That just made me feel worse!

(FEB 27, 2015) First outing since the procedure. We spend the afternoon at my father-in-law's. Rick calls before we arrive, to ask about lunch. His dad says he has some yogurt for me and sandwich fixings for him and Rick. I can't face the thought of more yogurt! We stop for a frozen dinner for me--cheese lasagna. It turns out to be a bit of a challenge to chew, but only around the edges where the cheese has baked to a hard crust. Our Chihuahua, Jack, is happy to take care of those for me.

For supper, my father-in-law makes us meatloaf with a mashed potato 'crust' - a recipe from his neighbor. Really good! And I have eaten meatloaf since my dentures, so I think this will be okay. The only problem I have is the onion chunks he has included in the meat mixture. They are still solid enough that it hurts to try to chew them. I just pick them out. It's a good recipe--one I will definitely save and recommend to other "teeth newbies"--but I would leave out the onions and substitute onion powder in their place. Still, the meal was a success, and I start to believe I may even be comfortable enough to eat out someday. Not sure when but – someday. I also ate a roll! I nearly wept, it was so good to eat bread again! I don't know why I hadn't tried bread before. I even bit off a small piece of it - with my side teeth. Everything I read says not to bite with my front teeth although I am not sure why.

At home I had chocolate, cream-filled, sandwich cookies. I broke them in half and soaked them in a mug of milk until they were soft. This was another treat I didn't expect to be able to eat for some time. And it was so simple. I just had to change my approach. If you can't do things the same way you used to - find a different way! I had read something online about a woman who was able to eat cookies by soaking them in milk. So simple. You don't have to leap tall buildings - just take the elevator. There is always another way.

Chewing still takes a lot of focus. The dentist only relined the upper teeth, so my lowers are not as tight. I was chewing a bite of meatloaf and potato on just one side. I know they tell you to chew on both sides to prevent shifting but it feels so awkward. My lower teeth slipped - it felt like they were totally off my gums. Bit of a panic there! I managed to maneuver them back into position and was more careful after that. No one else noticed so probably as long as you don't say anything, or do anything like take the teeth out, no one will realize.

So the lesson for the day? "Keep calm and take it one bite at a time!" When I was training for - I think every job I've ever had, there was always some variation of the same advice. "Fake it till you make it," the trainer would tell us. They would explain that, no matter how new or nervous we were, if we faked confidence, the customer would never know the difference. In that situation, like in this one, you really had no choice. There was no way to get from point A to point B without stepping out on faith. You had to keep reminding yourself - I can do this. With jobs, there were people to help. Supervisors, co-workers, you weren't out there alone.

Donna Wylie

A support system is just as important - maybe more so! - in this situation. Somebody's got to be there to remind you how far you have come. To celebrate the victories ("you ate pancakes!") and temper the failures ("crackers may hurt now, but last week you couldn't even manage pancakes. You'll get there!").

Week 4 and Beyond - Teeth truce

(FEB 28, 2015) Ordinary day. Errands, relaxing with a movie, playing games on my Kindle. Ordinary days are a kind of miracle in themselves. Gives me hope that someday all this 'stuff' in my mouth will be ordinary as well. Part of a routine. I have already gotten more comfortable with cleaning my teeth after eating.

My lips still feel chapped from the reline two days ago. After they do that process there is always a sticky residue on my mouth and around my lips. Almost like a glue. Here is where the support person comes in handy. The dentist just hands you a cup of water to rinse. Mouth-wash would be sooo much better! Anything to rinse the taste out. Water just doesn't cut it! Rick got me paper towels and directed me to a mirror on the wall behind me so I could see where the glue-like substance was that I could feel, just not wipe off. I had to scrape with my fingernails! It was a bit obsessive perhaps, but at that point I needed something else to focus on.

(MARCH 1, 2015) Ate crackers today. Buttery, round, easily conquered, crackers. I still break things up but I am slowly getting more used to eating with dentures. The challenge at present is the lowers. Keeping them in place. They are quite loose and have a tendency to raise up with the food. I am getting better at controlling them, and hope the permanent ones will be more obedient. I still struggle with depression. It's a kind of surreal feeling still, to know my teeth are gone forever. Rick is eating popcorn. The smell beckons me and I wonder...could I do it? Can I handle popcorn? I try a few kernels. YES!!! I can eat popcorn! Not fast but that's okay. Best part--if pesky kernels stick in my teeth, I can take the teeth out and rinse them! Whoo-Hoo!

(MARCH 2, 2015) Sounds senile - heck, maybe it Is - but I consider this a step forward. I stepped out of the shower today, saw my open, empty denture case and had a brief moment of 'oh-god-where-did-I-put-my-teeth' panic. The fact that they were in my mouth feels like a positive thing. For just the briefest moment, I forgot I had something 'foreign' in my mouth!

I think I am in the "contrary phase" of learning to eat. Rick remarked how all of a sudden, I am eating things I haven't been able to eat for the last month. Like hotdogs (no bun) and fries. And corn chips. "Don't worry", I joked, "I'm not biting off more than I can chew." Well.... maybe. My lower gums hurt a bit tonight. I need to slow it down a bit, perhaps.

Rick made scrambled eggs for breakfast. And fried tater tots. Little bit of a challenge to chew but I did it. The grease proved more than I could handle, however. Or perhaps it was my sudden switch to more normal food. Whatever it was, it triggered a nasty little payback from my lower intestine. I retreated to soothing comfort food. For lunch I had a cup of applesauce. I broke crackers into the cup - one cracker at a time so they wouldn't get soggy. This was a new combo for me. I often eat pudding on saltine crackers--I like the mix of sweet and salty, soft and crunchy. This was a nice variation. And the applesauce calmed my cranky tummy.

For supper we did fries and hotdogs. And then cake. And later, corn chips. There goes any weight I lost in the first 3 weeks of this denture diet! My eating has gone from "starve" to "gluttony" rather quickly. Hopefully this will even out once I get my fill of all the foods I haven't been able to eat this past month.

(MARCH 4, 2015) The fact that I am not recording notes each day is another indicator that things are slowly returning to routine. The only ongoing aggravation is the loose fit of the lowers. They often stick to what I am chewing and lift up. That will be solved to a great degree, once I have the permanent lowers. Meanwhile I am trying to look at it as good exercise for my jaw muscles, to get them used to gripping the teeth.

(AFTERNOON) Turned into kind of a blah day. We went to a Thrift store we had discovered by accident the previous week, anticipating another great 50% off treasure hunt. Nothing! Back at home, I discovered that potato chips are

Donna Wylie

Not easy to eat. I was sure it would be a breeze. Nice thin, crispy chips. Apparently thin doesn't necessarily equal easy. Guess I'll save potato chips for another time. I was able to eat corn chips one night - but those are thicker, easier to maneuver in my mouth. I don't know why I feel so bothered by 'chip failure'....

When I think about it, I realize I have been modifying my diet for years. My teeth have been bad for a long time. I started losing them 30 years ago when I was in my 30's. I used to joke about how "the warranty ran out when I hit 21" adding "had I known I was going to live so long I would have gotten the extended plan!" But it was no laughing matter.

My whole family has problems with their teeth. I remember my older sister having to choose soft foods, like pancakes, when we went out to lunch with our aunt. She was too ashamed to say anything, but later admitted to me that she had a number of loose teeth. My brothers and younger sister have all had issues as well. We grew up in a time before fluoride, which probably wouldn't have mattered anyway, since we grew up on a farm with well water. We also didn't go to the dentist. It was too expensive with six children. I remember getting my teeth cleaned once a year when the dental hygienist came to our rural school. That was the closest we came to regular dental care. I'm not criticizing - just giving background. No one nagged us to brush our teeth every night, though we all understood we should. I know another factor that contributed to our weak teeth was the 'milk' we drank. I put that word in quotes because I don't consider that beverage to be milk. It was powdered milk that my mom would mix with water. Or Try to mix. There were always lumps at the bottom. And the taste was something even cows wouldn't recognize! So even if it had all the important nutrients, it wouldn't have mattered because we did anything we could to avoid drinking it!

(**MARCH 5 & 6, 2015**) Feeling yucky. Hover flu. Hangs over me but never lands.

(**MARCH 8, 2015**) Progressing. I'm almost at tortilla chips stage. Still hurts a bit to chew such thin, hard things. Corn chips are easier. Going to try pizza for lunch, so I only ate 1 corn chip. When Rick asked if I wanted more I replied "no, I'm saving myself for pizza."

Stop the presses! I ate PIZZA! It was one of those cheap, limp, frozen things. Rick joked that he wouldn't necessarily call that pizza. I told him it's certainly closer than I've gotten in the last month!! I had to cut it into bite-sized pieces, and it was still a challenge but...the point is.... I ATE PIZZA! Whoot! Whoot! Happy dance! Jack helped by volunteering to eat the hard crust bits that I just couldn't conquer.

(**LATER THAT SAME DAY**) My confidence crashes again when I try to eat supper. We are having boxed meal helper; potatoes in a stroganoff sauce;

Donna Wylie

one of my favorites. Rick asks if I can eat that. "Sure!", I say, still full of pizza confidence. After all, potatoes shouldn't be a challenge, right? Wrong again! Though the potatoes are well cooked and tender, there is something about the shape (slices) that I just can't seem to chew. My bottom plate is a temporary and very loose but generally controllable. Not this time. A bit of potato sneaks underneath my teeth, creating an opening for bits of ground turkey to follow. Mouth mutiny!

It's the first time since I got dentures, that I totally lost control of my lower plate! Nothing to do but retire to the bathroom where I restore order. Rick obligingly chops up my supper. He's getting really good at this by now. Backwards slide. At least that's what it feels like. My inner voice pokes fun. "First day with yer new teeth, Vern?" I admit defeat - for now. But... I ate PIZZA!

(MARCH 9, 2015) sliced things are going to be a challenge. Snacking on crackers and slices of my favorite cheese - Vermont sharp white cheddar. Thinly sliced seems hard to control so I fold a slice to make 3 layers. Nope - too thick. My still healing gums protest. I try just 2 layers and have a little better luck, but the whole process of eating seems like a wrestling match' My cough - whatever it is - has returned and I am feeling draggy and discouraged. Woke up once last night with a jaw ache. Right at the hinge part, under my ears. I know my mouth is working hard to adapt to these new teeth, but I'm getting that panicky irrational feeling. Like I just want to scream "get these things out of my mouth!" and go back to the way things were. I know that's not possible, or reasonable, it's just visceral. Some days I just don't want to be on this ride....

I long for normal food - pumpkin pie. And lemon meringue pie; and oh! - chocolate silk pie. Those are probably doable. I'd also like my favorite breakfast meal - toast and peanut butter with canned peaches and cinnamon sugar on top. That might be a challenge. Or would it? Lately the things I think Should be easy are Not. My world feels turned upside down, my emotions on a runaway roller coaster ride. It's exhausting.

(MARCH 11, 2015) Mmmmmm-milky way bars! They melt in your mouth, no chewing required. Good thing because I was feeling too lazy to go get my teeth!

(MARCH 12, 2015) Feels like I'm stuck at the "Food is a Bother" stage. I'm tired of having to put so much thought into eating. It's been 5 weeks since I got dentures and I'm losing my patience and my sense of humor.. Lord give me strength!

(MARCH 13, 2015) I now have a whole new interpretation of the phrase "my jaw dropped". This is why you always cover your mouth when you yawn!

Donna Wylie

(**M**arch **14, 2015**) I get impatient and angry and try to eat "normal" food. As a result, my jaws ache and I get frustrated and depressed. I'm having Cream of Wheat and orange juice for breakfast. Giving myself and my teeth a rest!

(**M**arch **15, 2015**) The debate continues - teeth in or out at night? My dentist says I should take them out. My dad-in-law says that's not practical because I still have 2 of my natural teeth, canines, on the bottom and I might bite myself. It's true - those teeth are quite sharp. Then there are the people who say don't ever take them out because you won't be able to get them back in! There's too much conflicting information out there!

(**M**arch **16, 2015**) I'm slowly learning how to bite. For lunch I had ham salad on one of those soft Hawaiian sweet rolls. The ham salad was my own concoction; just ham, a little celery salt, a bit of sweet relish and enough mayonnaise to make it an acceptable texture. I cut the roll in half - starting small. It was delicious! The taste of victory!

Afterwards, we went and got a soft ice cream cone, and I ate it cone and all! Takes forever, and made my jaw ache but it gives me hope. Eventually, I will be done with all this healing and adjusting. I will survive to chew again!

Denture Adventure

(**MARCH 19, 2015**) I've been thinking. WHY should dentures be such a shameful secret? It's time to admit the truth--not everyone's teeth last a lifetime. Time to open your mouth and be counted! Denture wearers Unite! It's time to come out of the closet! Er--plastic cup. Er glass... Another reline appointment. Never gets any easier from my point of view, although my husband says I am handling it way better than the first time. The doctor still says it will be 6 months until things are completely healed to the point that I can go a couple years between adjustments.

The 6-month mark is when I will get my temporary lowers replaced with the permanent set. So - another 4 1/2 months. I just have to be patient, they said. No other choice, I said. One day, one step, one bite at a time.

(**MARCH 20, 2015**) I ate Barbecue! Yes, the pulled pork was Ultra tender, melt-in-your-mouth good. But there were sides, too - macaroni salad, barbecue beans and fried onion strings. I ate them all! And a roll. Life is starting to return to normal. Barbecue is a great motivator! I think I'm ready for lobster.

MARCH 21, 2015) Benefit of dentures – I am able to slice a giant pan of onions without a single tear! Rick's eyes were watering from yards away, and usually I would be crying, but not this time. I could feel a slight burning in the back of my throat but that was it!

(MARCH 25, 2015) Just when I'm thinking things are starting to return to normal, I have a "gaggy day."Everyone heals differently. Seems like common sense, but it's easy to get caught up in peer pressure, even with dentures. Especially with dentures, I think! This is a new experience, and it's natural to want reassurance that every-thing is going along as it should. Word of advice - get a professional opinion if you have concerns.

(MARCH 27, 2015) What everyone says is true - the uppers are easier to keep in place than the lowers. That seems to defy the law of gravity. My father-in-law says it's because of the suction. Is he saying my head is a vacuum?

(APRIL 4, 2015) So, am I the only one who has never used denture adhesive? I've had these things for two months now, and it still feels like I don't know how to work them! There needs to be one of those "Dummies" guides for dentures!

(APRIL 8, 2015) Tried denture adhesive for the first time. Sea-Bond wafers on the lowers, Poligrip paste on the top. Doing a comparison. My father-in-law gave me some sample packs to try. Doesn't take long to decide. The paste feels too much like the reline material and triggers an immediate gag (panic) attack. The wafers are better, soft and comfortable and easier to remove at the end of the day. I'm sold. No need for exten-sive testing. I keep the tube of paste, however, for times when I need the teeth to stay 'glued' in

Denture Adventure

place.

(APRIL 11, 2015) There are days when I feel like I am back at the beginning again and I feel discouraged. It helps to look back sometimes, to see how far I have climbed. I can rest a minute. Not every day needs conquering.

(APRIL 12, 2015) Still have a tiny sharp bit in one of my tooth sockets. Bone working its way out, according to the dentist. Kind of a pain - literally! Feels like a real mild toothache. This is another aspect of dentures I wasn't aware of. A friend tells me she had bits of bone working their way to the surface for months after her procedure also. Why does no one tell you these things?

(APRIL 16, 2015) I have discovered that even adhesive wafers will break down into nasty, glue-y bits. Maybe I had them on wrong? Maybe I shouldn't have used
lowers on my uppers? This is still all so trial and (mostly) error. I tried the full uppers wafer one day - actually made my teeth feel looser! Like I had a - you know - blanket between the roof of my mouth and the upper plate. I thought maybe a more custom fit was the solution. So I cut down some lower wafers I had, and lined just the sides and a strip at the back of the upper plate. Kind of similar to the way the paste tells you to apply it.

Worked great! Until...... I took them out some 7-8 hours later. And the wafer was a gluey, sticky

mess. Jeez! Maybe I do need more field testing.
(APRIL 17, 2015) Think one of my biggest
reliefs was when I found out I could still indulge
in my favorite habit of ice-chewing! .... it's the
little things...

(APRIL 19, 2015) There are times when I forget
I have teeth in my mouth .... sounds like a line
from a Dr. Seuss book!

(APRIL 22, 2015) Just because you Can, doesn't
mean you have to. Some days I just don't feel like
chewing!

(APRIL 28, 2015) Ate a chicken rice bowl from
one of our favorite take-out restaurants - plenty
of veggies, which I love. BUT....they do them the
'healthy' way. You know, just barely cooked, to
preserve all their veggie-goodness. Which meant
it was a real "teeth-test"! I handled it, though. Just
shows how far I've come in (almost) 3 months!

(APRIL 30, 2015) That moment when you
order a sausage McMuffin, then remember the
last time you had one was when you had your
own teeth! Good thing I'm in my "defiant" phase.
I conquer the breakfast sandwich!

(MAY 2, 2015) I ate a peanut butter and jelly
sandwich!! I was worried about how I'd handle
"sticky foods." But, hey PB&J is a requirement for
a balanced life! It wasn't as hard as I thought it
would be. The bread helped keep the peanut

butter from coming in direct contact with my dentures. I felt triumphant; one more item marked off my (lunch) bucket list!

(MAY 4, 2015) My father-in-law Really wanted me to try eating corn on the cob. As I told him, my preference has always been to cut it off the cob, even when I had teeth. More corn, less mess. And OK, let's be honest--all that butter just slides off the cob! Such a waste!

(MAY 6, 2015) Today I ate licorice! Black, fat chunks each about 2" long. Chewy but manage-able. Another food group conquered. Sounds silly, but fellow "falsie-wearers" (teeth, of course) can relate, I'm sure. Next up.... lettuce!, which they say is difficult. So I've been avoiding it. That's wrong. I can't let food scare me!

(MAY 11, 2015) It's weird, the things I miss now that I have dentures. Like being able to bite my nails. Well, I suppose that's one way to break a bad habit!

(MAY 13, 2015) You know you are getting used to dentures when you accidentally start to brush your teeth.

(MAY 17, 2015) I ate PIZZA! Pizzeria Pizza. Okay, I had to cut it up, but I ate it! First time I've had real pizza in months! It was heavenly!

(MAY 19, 2015) Had one of my favorite "pre-D"

treats yesterday - a pretzel bagel! Love to warm them in the microwave for a few seconds and then dip them in mustard. Mmmmm! I am learning almost any food is a food I can eat, with some minor changes. Rather than biting the bagel, I tore off bite-sized pieces. I'm thinking apples are possible using the same principle. Can probably even dip the bites in caramel dip.

(MAY 29, 2015) Really need to get in and get my teeth adjusted. Dreading the thought but it must be done.

(JUNE 2, 2015) Adjustment went okay. Better than last time, according to my "denture co-pilot", Rick. I tried a few techniques from my previous research, as well as some new ones I'd read about. So far acupressure seems to work best for me.

(JUNE 16, 2015) Another day when I feel like I have chopsticks in my mouth. Chewing feels awkward and unfamiliar. I know this too shall pass, but some days I grow weary of this process.

(JUNE 19, 2015) Ever get a hair in your mouth? Used to hate that. Could feel it in there, just couldn't find the little bugger! Now I can just take my teeth out and have a closer look.

(JUNE 24, 2016) I've been thinking. Why not nuts? Caramel I understand - because of course I had to test it myself. It came as no surprise when caramel won that skirmish by gluing itself to my dentures I'm still plotting my revenge!) So what is it about nuts? Too hard? But I'm still able to crunch ice.... Might damage the teeth? My contrary nature demands explanation. A-googling I go!

(JUNE 26, 2015) Some days I just don't feel like chewing.... think I've slid back into Stage 5. This too shall pass, I realize, but I wasn't prepared for this 6-month roller coaster! Be sure you have a support person (I call them "denture buddies") or group of people.

(JUNE 27, 2015) Aw, Nuts! The only information I could find online is either how nuts are something I shouldn't eat, or vague comments about how nuts are "difficult" to eat. What the heck?! I'm not looking to crack walnuts with my teeth, people! I just want to eat a cashew! Maybe a pecan. And - dare I hope? - a brazil nut?

(JULY 4, 2015) I did it! I ate nuts! Cashews. Oh yum!! I used the same technique as other food - chew with the back teeth, food divided between both sides of the mouth. The field test was Deliciously successful!

(JULY 10, 2015) Little less than 1 week to my next appointment. Getting nervous already. Just Hate the gagging part! Checking my supplies - accu-pressure wrist bands, throat spray, music.

Hopefully they work.

(JULY 16, 2015) Reline day. I thought. The dentist didn't even do anything today. When I went into the office, the receptionist asked what I was having done that day. I said I had no idea, I thought I was there for a fitting for my permanent lowers. No one seemed to know anything about it. Another error on their part. Or miscommunication. Whatever the reason, it's frustrating! I wasted all that worry for nothing! Next appointment August 5th - my 6-month anniversary and time (finally!) for the permanent teeth. The dentist gal told me that they will do the impressions for my permanent teeth when I come in Aug 5th. I immediately thought of the gag-awful 1st experience with impressions.

The panic must have shown on my face because she hurried to reassure me, saying it was just like the relines only the material didn't taste bad. I nodded and said "oh Sure! Save the good stuff for the end. Right before the Yelp review!" She looked a little worried, until she realized I was joking.

(AUG 5, 2015) The fitting for my permanent lower plate went well. As Carrie promised, the material they used didn't taste bad. It was a wax kind of substance, that I bit down on just for a few minutes. Didn't even need all my stress gear! They put a metal plate in my mouth – the base for the permanent teeth.

Denture Adventure

Everyone had a look and declared it good.

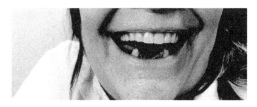

(Aug 7, 2015) Unplanned trek to the dentist this morning. My upper teeth were making my mouth really sore. I called and left a message for the dentist, even though I was afraid it would mean another round of goopy gunk. But, all the dentist did was grind down and smooth the plates a bit. It made a Huge difference!

(Aug 17, 2015) There are times when I am more aware that I have teeth in my mouth...I know I'm sounding like a Dr. Seuss rhyme again, but it's hard to explain. What I mean is, some-times my dentures feel "foreign"; even after 6 months. It's like having a hair in your mouth. Only bigger. Sigh. Nothing I can't work (or in this case, chew) around.

(Aug 24, 2015) Under the "not fun" category - Fighting through an hour of expressway traffic, to get to the dentist, just so they can test the lower plate framework in my mouth. Think FedEx would have been faster! However, it's a Good visit when the worst part about going to the dentist - is the Commute!

Donna Wylie

(Aug 27, 2015) My New (permanent) smile.

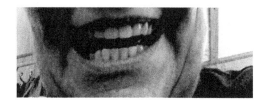

(Aug 28, 2015) Slight - okay, major - panic last night when I couldn't get my new lower plate out. Hyperventilating now, just thinking about it! ...Breathe!..I just needed a slight adjustment.

(Sept 1, 2015) Note to self - in an emergency, Cheetos make an Excellent glue! Unless...the emergency happens to be that you have Cheetos stuck All over your dentures! Live and learn!

(Sept 2, 2015) Still getting used to my "new" bottom plate partials. There is a metal "halter" kind of thing that fits over my two remaining bottom teeth, and help anchor the partials in place. Very solid. Also very painful! So I end up taking them out after about a half day, and reverting back to my temporary teeth. The dentist said these may require a "couple adjustments". Just when I thought SEVEN months of dental visits, adjustments and gagging was coming to an end (finally!). I'm telling you, it's enough to try anyone's patience!

Denture Adventure

(Sept 3, 2015) Yesterday at the dentist, I got my lowers adjusted. When the girl gave them back, of course she asked how they felt. I told her they felt Much better, no longer rubbing. She said, "try moving your mouth like you're eating. See if that feels ok." I replied, "you know, I think if you gave me an egg McMuffin it would be easier to check if it feels okay to eat...." She just laughed. Pretty sure I wasn't kidding.

(Sept 4, 2015)
Denture discussion with my husband:

Donna: I bit my tongue yesterday
Rick: With your New teeth? That wasn't nice.
Donna: I know! They need an adjustment (pause)...An Attitude adjustment!

(Sept 7, 2015) Mmmmm! Pretzel bagel! My favorite! Practical application of the phrase "bit off more than I could chew"! I need to remember to take smaller bites.

(Sept 14, 2015) Ever bite the inside of your mouth? Then keep doing it? Probably because that area is swollen. Or my teeth hate me. Yeah. I still think they need an attitude adjustment. Wonder if my dentist can do that...?

(Sept 18, 2015) Think I insulted my dentist. I went in to have cavities filled in my two remaining teeth. The dentist gave me some shots to numb the area and left for a few minutes to allow the Novocaine time to take effect. When he came back, he asked if I was numb. It didn't feel like I expected--you know, like when your jaw feels all fuzzy and fat? So I said I didn't know, and asked, "how can you tell when it's numb enough?" He said something about how "when you've done thousands of these," you just know. Oops. I'm sure my comment had nothing to do with how the procedure hurt. Pretty sure...Maybe... I then moved to the hygienist for deep cleaning and scraping under the gum-line. Which included the use of a laser to remove dead tissue. It didn't hurt, just smelled like something burning. Which it was, I guess. Me! So--Not my best visit, to say the least.

(SEPT 27, 2015) Hard to remember (or don't want to!) those first weeks days of mush food!

(SEPT 29, 2015) Dentist appointment tomorrow. More "deep cleaning" (shudder!). Gonna have them adjust the lowers. I've got a blister-like sore on one side of my mouth where they must be rubbing. Why hasn't anyone come up with a more pliable material for the base? I hate when my mouth hurts!

(OCT 5, 2015) So the deep cleaning wasn't all that bad. Not fun, definitely, just - not bad. She used spray lidocaine to numb my gums. Nasty taste! Once again I wonder why they can't make better tasting dental products! They know we are putting this ____ in our mouths, right???!!! Sorry; feeling sick and cranky today

Denture Adventure

(Oct 6, 2015) Denture lesson # 215 - it is advisable to remove dentures Prior to swallowing foul tasting cough syrup, as the liquid will work its way under the plates in order to linger as long as possible on your palate.

(Oct 7, 2015) Under the category of "things I Never imagined myself saying (Ever!)":
"Hang on, let me get my teeth"
Another lesson learned - if I am feeling nauseous, dentures seem to make it worse.

(Oct 16, 2015) My teeth bit me! Sorry for the extreme close up, but it's a bit hard to see (left side in photo). It was bleeding like crazy last night!

Be warned, denture-wearers. These teeth bite!

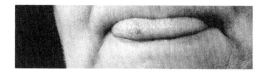

(Oct 23, 2015) There was a positive outcome from biting my tongue. I am more relaxed about eating. After all, I Know these things can handle biting food!

(Oct 27, 2015) Dentist appointment tomorrow. More poking and cleaning of my 2 remaining teeth. Last time...I hope...please! Been going for one thing or another since February.

Donna Wylie

(Nov 2, 2015) Note to self. Cornmeal is powerful stuff. One tiny little grain can dive under the bottom plate and make eating a nightmare! Shades of "princess and the pea"!

(Nov 12, 2015) Sometimes I put my dentures in, go strolling out of the bathroom and - WHAM!! Surprise gag reflex! I can usually regain control right away - deep breath and determination.
Other times, I have to remove the uppers until my salivary glands and I calm down. It's almost like a mini flashback to all those dental visits when I would end up teary-eyed and tired from fighting my gag-reflex.

Much as I hated those times, they taught me valuable lessons. Like how to focus on breathing. Count the minutes. Walk in place. Visualize my happy place. Coping skills.
There's something good that comes from every bad experience.

(Nov 19, 2015) Dear dentists - Please, please, please let us know what you are doing! We realize, this may be routine to you but it's all brand-new and scary to us. Help us out!

(Dec 3, 2015) Still haven't figured out a way to eat caramels with dentures. There should be attachments you can get to deal with different types of food. You know. Like vacuum cleaner attachments.

Denture Adventure

(DEC 23, 2015) Holy mainstream, Batman! I've discovered denture Toothpaste! It was soooo satisfying to be able to brush my teeth! Okay, so I was holding them in my hand while I did that, but still...!

(DEC 28, 2015) Blindsided by candy! I thought fudge would be safe. But no! It's nearly as deadly as caramel as far as stickiness.
Biting it started a tug of war game between the fudge and my teeth. I eventually won but this is not a treat to be enjoyed in public. On the plus side, removable teeth do make it possible to lick every drop of sticky chocolaty goodness from them. But I will deny that if asked.

(FEB 7, 2016) Feb 5th was also the 1 year "birthday" of my dentures. Happy birthday, teeth!

(FEB 12, 2016) I don't know why, but I immediately distrust people with overly white teeth....
I know everyone is doing those teeth whitening procedures lately, I just find the color.... disturbing....

(FEB 24, 2016) That moment when you realize...the most expensive thing you're wearing is your teeth.

(MARCH 10, 2016) I still get days when my teeth gag me. I'm kind of an expert at gagging now but it still frustrates me.

Donna Wylie

(MARCH 24, 2016) I wonder if I will ever have complete control over my gag reflex. My dentures still make me gag. Not every time, just once in a while, which actually is worse - I never see it coming! Been experimenting with various techniques. Warm water rinse, cool water rinse. Breathe through my nose, deep breathing to calm my body. Clamping my jaws shut. Hard to tell if something is working or not, until the gag happens.

(MAY 4, 2016) I hate it when my dentures make me gag. I think of my dad-in-law saying it's just mind over matter. So I get angry at myself. And that turns into determination. I Will conquer you, evil gag reflex!
or.... maybe I will just take the teeth out. And let them sit in their little case. In the dark. And think about what they've done.
Yeah! That will teach them!

(MAY 6, 2016) I've turned into this weird teeth-fetish kind of freak. The other day, I was talking to a fellow teacher and suddenly, I just had to know...
"Are those your teeth?", I asked. I had the weirdest urge to reach out and tug on them, like a little kid pulling on Santa's beard.
Yep. Teeth Envy. Probably a 12-step program for that somewhere.

Denture Adventure

It just takes one bite of caramel to remind me why I no longer eat them. One blissful, dark chocolate, Milky Way bite.
Sometimes I forget.

(MAY 15, 2016) My dad-in-law is still trying to get me to eat corn on the cob! He serves it every time we go over there for dinner. Thing is, I've always cut mine off the cob. Never liked the way the butter kept sliding off the ear of corn, or how greasy my hands would get. So, really, I have no incentive to try to eat corn off the cob.
Now if he'd been serving Milky Way or Snickers bars, that would have been a different story! Sigh.
I miss caramel.

(MAY 22, 2016) Been re-reading this journal. I had almost forgotten how long it took to eat "real" food again after my dental procedure.
When I was researching online, all the sites talked about eating soft foods for the first week, and then adding in harder food, avoiding things like nuts. Made it sound like you only had to tolerate 1 week of gelatin and yogurt.

Wrong! It's a Very gradual process, stretching over weeks. That's why I believe the recipe book I'm compiling is so important. One of my favorite recipes in that book, is a chocolate-peanut butter-butterscotch shake. It's made with protein powder and tastes heavenly! My sister turned me on to protein powder when I was searching for more nutritious food. I was reluctant to try it – how could it taste good if it was good for you, right? But my body needed protein and vitamins to heal, so I gave it a try.

Denture Adventure

Here is that recipe, for you to try:

Chocolate Peanut-Butterscotch Smoothie – My Favorite!
1 cup milk (any kind)
½ - ¾ cup cold water
1 cup ice cubes
1 scoop chocolate protein powder
1 large Tablespoon peanut butter
1 Tablespoon butterscotch instant pudding, dry mix
Put everything in the blender and process until well
mixed. Makes one giant portion or two human-sized
ones. Enjoy!

Final (for now) Thoughts:

I've been trying to think of a way to end this book; a "conclusion", if you will. But unlike fiction or finite non-fiction, this saga will continue. At some point down the road, my dentures will need adjusting and refitting. I also may eventually lose the two anchor teeth I have left on the bottom, which would necessitate a full lower plate and everything that entails. My father-in-law has implants that his lower teeth attach to.

They look like tiny screws that are embedded in your jaw bone. The very idea makes me shudder! But the main lesson I have learned from this whole process is – I am stronger than my fear. Whatever happens, whatever new challenges come my way in the future, I will abide. So there may come a time when I feel a need to share another "denture adventure" with you all. Until then – stay calm and chew on!

Made in United States
North Haven, CT
01 December 2022

27661093R00036